The Magic of Marigolds

Marigolds for Health and Beauty

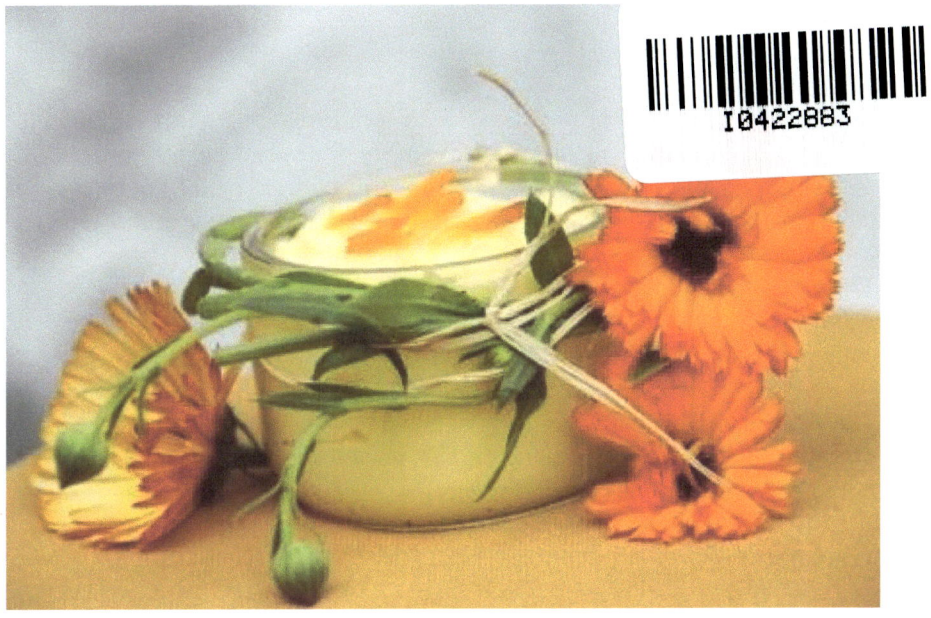

Dueep J Singh

Natural Remedy Series

Mendon Cottage Books

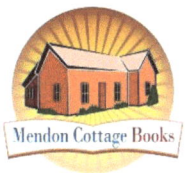

JD-Biz Publishing

Disclaimer

The information is this book is provided for informational purposes only. It is not intended to be used and medical advice or a substitute for proper medical treatment by a qualified health care provider. The information is believed to be accurate as presented based on research by the author.

The contents have not been evaluated by the U.S. Food and Drug Administration or any other Government or Health Organization and the contents in this book are not to be used to treat cure or prevent disease.

The author or publisher is not responsible for the use or safety of any diet, procedure or treatment mentioned in this book. The author or publisher is not responsible for errors or omissions that may exist.

Warning

The Book is for informational purposes only and before taking on any diet, treatment or medical procedure it is recommended to consult with your primary health care provider.

Our books are available at

1. Amazon.com

2. Barnes and Noble

3. Itunes

4. Kobo

5. Smashwords

6. Google Play Books

Table of Contents

Introduction

I was under the impression that the beautiful Marigold was just an ornamental flower looking great in my garden, until I found out that it was an herbaceous perennial, used in herbal medicines, natural remedies, and also in beauty recipes. So, this book is going to tell you all about the magic of marigolds, how to see them grow and flourish in your garden, and also use them in cookery, as well as in beauty recipes.

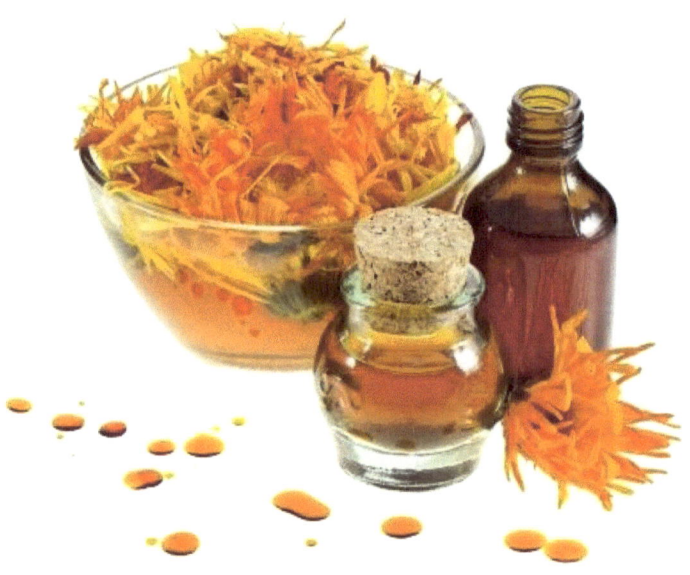

In Asia, marigolds are an integral part of social life. Every auspicious ceremony needs garlands of marigolds and jasmines to adorn the houses, photographs of the gods, goddesses, and guests who have been invited to bless the ceremony with their presence. Marigolds are originally natives of

North India, Africa, and Mexico. From here, they were taken all over the civilized world by traders.

So that means you are going to see Calendula officinalis, otherwise known as garden Marigold , common Marigold and even pot Marigold , growing all in warm and temperate regions all over the globe. But a Mexican priest told me that ancient legend says the name Marigold is supposed to be in praise of the Virgin Mary – "Mary's Gold". Also, he told me that this flower named *cempasúchil* in Mexico was considered to be the sacred flower of the dead, and had to be offered during the celebration of The Day of the Dead, when people prayed to their departed near and dear ones.

In India, this flower is called *Satvarga- just like the Sun.*

Marigolds may bloom throughout the year, if the conditions are favorable, and the sun is warm and shining, so naturally this flower is one of the most preferred choices to use in happy celebrations, when you want to depict and praise light and sunshine.

Do you know that the ancient Greeks, Romans, Egyptians and Indians used Marigold flowers as a natural dye? They also colored foods with Marigold flowers to give the dish a golden yellow tint, especially when they did not have turmeric or saffron around.

So if you want to nibble Marigolds, remember that only Pot Marigold Species T. tenuifolia florets are edible. Do not use Marigold leaves in any culinary masterpiece.

Use of Marigolds in Herbal Lore And Tradition

The pungent and bitter odor of the flower is due to essential oils and saponins which are very useful as antifungals and antioxidants. The yellow orange color is due to carotenoids. Many popular Marigold varieties include the deep orange Alpha, the bright yellow Sun Glow and Jane Harmony, and other orange, yellow and orange – red varieties like Orange Prince and Indian Prince .

There are many amusing myths which are connected to the flower. In India, if you presented somebody with a garland of Marigolds, it meant that you were ready to be his friend and he had to take the offer in the manner it was given. One of my friends who is interested in Wicca told me that marigolds were used by witches to cast spells, to protect somebody and to bring luck, happiness, peace of mind, prosperity, success and love to anybody who wished for it. (Seems to be a pretty comprehensive and detailed list of all human aspirations hidden in one little flower, isn't it!)

It seems that if I added to Marigold flowers to my bath water it would bring me respect and admiration. That is why it seems that the ancient baths of Indian and other Asian royalty were always perfumed with Jasmine, rose and Marigold flowers.

And that is why I laughed, when she told me that young girls in ancient times went to the wise women and asked them for love lotions and love potions to attract the men of their choice. And the major ingredient of these potions was always marigolds.

Well, I being the perennial cynic, have the scientific explanation for this particular belief. It is just plain common sense, which the wise people of yore knew. Marigold is antifungal. If I have a bath in Marigold water, I will not suffer from skin diseases or body odor. Washing my mouth and face with Marigold   meant that I would not be suffering from halitosis and my face would have a rich squeaky clean glow. I would also have a clear, rich and glowing skin so dear to the heart of every young human. That means people would not flee my presence singing "here arrives, Stinky, Smelly, Grimy, again."

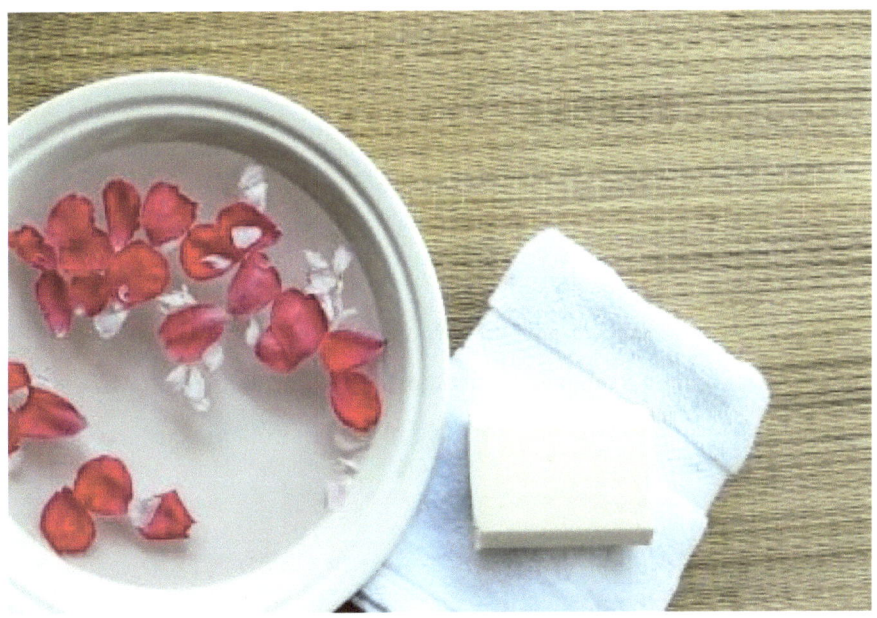

But why not? After all life is for living emperor size!

And that also means I would be the object of universal appreciation and envy [depending on gender] , because people who found somebody else ponging away due to the neglecting of daily ablutions would naturally gravitate into my sweeter smelling, well-scrubbed vicinity. Or perhaps make a beeline to the wise woman of the woods.

And so, when young ladies went to witches to ask for love potions and beauty lotions, a little bit of psychological lessons on basic   hygiene of regular bathing with an exotic ingredient of a mystic flower, made sure that the suitors came, saw and were conquered. No wonder these women trained in herbal lore were known as wise women.

Another belief is that Marigolds picked at early morning and noon strengthen and comfort the heart. As I positively love giving explanations which explain the reasons behind these beliefs, early morning and noon is the time when they are the most pungent, in order to attract insects. Anybody smelling marigolds picked at that time cannot go into hysterical or dainty swooning fits, because they act as powerful smelling salts. So, if a female happened to be neurotic, a good sniff of marigolds would soon bring her to her senses and would soon bring her out of her fit of temperamental behavior. So the next time you have somebody going into hysterics or swoons in your presence, pluck a Marigold out of a nearby vase instead of removing a ponging leather shoe [another well-known remedy for fits, swoons and hysteria]. Apply to nose and have the swooning one whooping awake double quick.

Elementary, my dear Watson!

Planting Marigolds In Your Garden

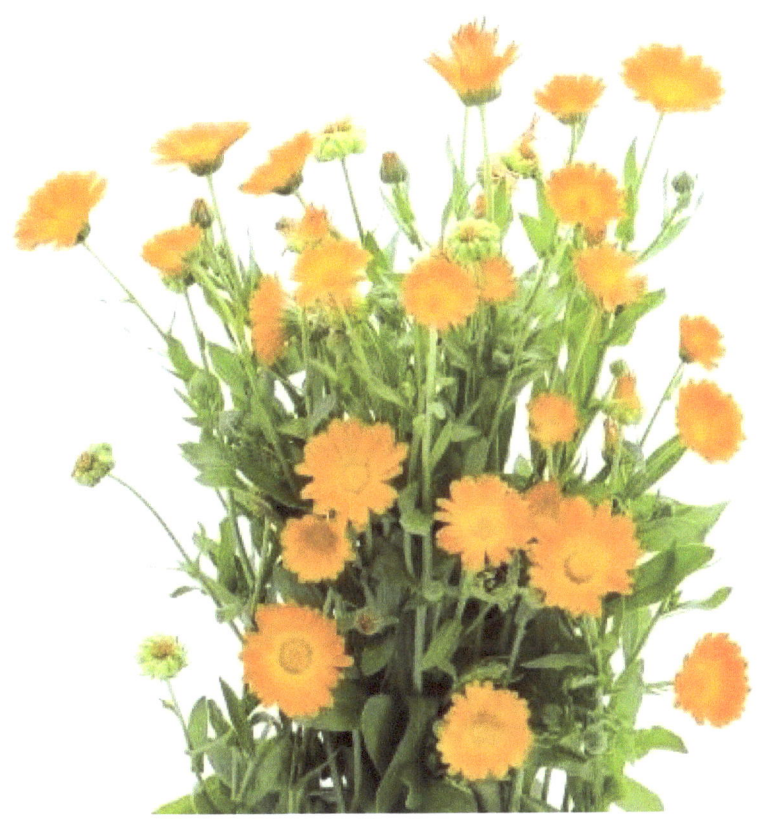

    I heard a gardener say that he planted marigolds in his garden, among his vegetables because it repelled pests and insects. Sorry, no, he was wrong. That is not true. Marigolds may get rid of many of the Nematode worms in the soil, but they do not repel harmful pests and insects in your garden. So the idea of interspersing your vegetable seeds with Marigold seeds is not something which I would advise. Besides, marigolds looks so good among the flowers. So why have them among the vegetables too?

When Is the Best Time to Plant Marigolds?

I would suggest that marigolds be planted as soon as the frost is over. If you have marigolds seeds leftover from last year's harvest, well and good, otherwise get seedlings from your nearby nursery.

Plant these seedlings, 12 – 24 inches apart. Marigolds are considered to be one of the most hardiest and easily maintained of all garden plants. That is why many lazy gardeners go in for planting marigolds on borders, in beds, and in every empty available garden space. That is because they do not need watering every day and you can water them only when you see that the bed is dry. Marigolds are planted in tropical regions in the first week of March so that the blooms are ready during the spring Festivals in April and May.

If you want to start seedlings from seed, plant them in a well-mulched bed until your seedlings are ready. I normally use mild organic fertilizer instead of strong chemical fertilizers. Besides, marigolds do not enjoy very heavily fertilized seed beds. The plants are going to be planted in a half shady and half sunny area. Once they start blooming, remove the dead flowers so that other flowers have plenty of space to grow.

Marigolds do not flourish in a region which is extremely hot or cold. But if you live in a mildly sunny mildly cool temperate region, you are going to get intoxicated with the strong smell of marigolds throughout the year. Some people consider this matter to be very strong and bitter. But as I said, that is because of their essential oils, which are extremely useful in Marigold creams and lotions.

If you want to grow marigolds in pots, that can also be done as long as the pots are placed in the shade.

Marigolds prefer sandy loamy and Clay soil. So, plant them in soil which is well-drained. Flowers are going to appear within 4 to 6 weeks of sowing.

Marigolds, alas, do not flourish in a moist and rainy climate. That is because the petals get soggy, waterlogged and starts to rot. That is the reason why I used to feel surprised as a child living in the mountains – where it rained every day – that our gardener used to plant lilies, gladioli, nasturtiums and other annual and perennial plants, but I never saw marigolds there until I came down to the plains, where the sun shone bright. Marigolds planted in the mountains and in moist climates are more prone to root rot, mildew and even mold.

How to collect seeds from your marigolds?

When you are ready to collect seeds for next years' sowing, you need to stop removing the flowers from the stalks. Wait till they are dried and brown. Just collect the flowers, pinch the dried ends between two fingers and give a hefty pull. The seeds which are black, thin, and pointy are going to fall out naturally. The seeds have to be stored in a dry and cool place ready for replanting next year. This is of course for places which are subject to heavy snow in the winter. In temperate regions gardeners just sow the seeds in prepared beds for them to come up next year in spring.

Beauty Products Made from Marigolds and Tips

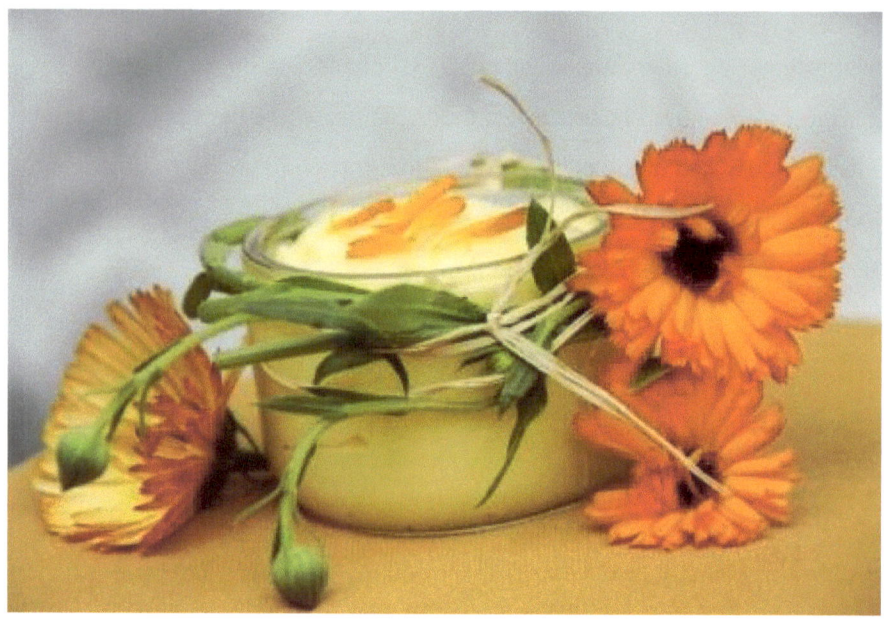

One fine morning I heard a colleague oohing and aahing over a really miraculous, really expensive, exotic branded skin product, and it had some magic, natural product in it, which made all the difference. Not being a botanist already gardener herself, she kept praising this amazing product, *Calendula*. When I told her that it was just the common garden Marigold, she was rather disappointed. And I felt bad, for having burst her bubble and pride in having bought something full of one "natural" magic ingredient and many chemical preservatives and fillers with limited shelf life at highly inflated prices. And then she asked me whether I used it in making my own personal beauty products. And when I said yes, she did not talk to me for one full day, because why had I kept my mouth shut about Calendula being the other name for Marigold?

So if my dear friend J. has the time to make beauty products using calendula, here they are, along with beauty tips and this is for you too, dear reader.

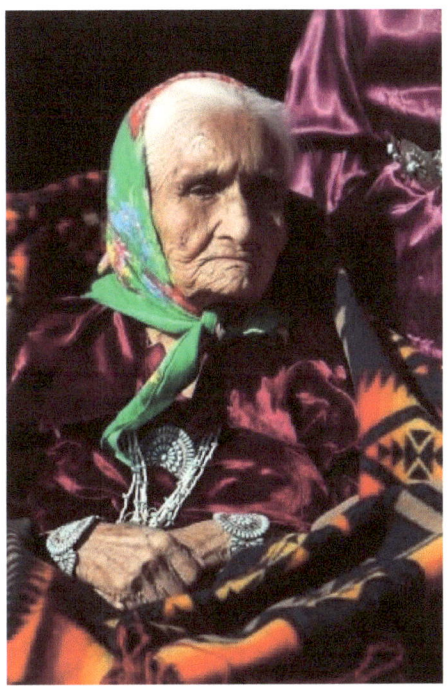

Now this wise old Navajo lady would know about Calendula and its properties through ancient tribal lore.

- Many beauty products have this secret ingredient placed in them and packaged attractively. I normally use the calendula petals of the short plant – the French Calendula –, because I find it more strong and potent.

- Anybody who is suffering from pimples should steep some of its petals into water, and place it in the Sun for three days. Remember to cover it, otherwise you might find some unnecessary ingredients like dust etc.

joining your Marigold water. Skim off the topmost layer of the water, which might have some petals floating upon it. This yellow colored water is the best refreshing skin lotion which gives a really golden glow to the skin. If you have any pimples, they really clear up with Marigold water baths. I normally put this Marigold water in my purse, and once I reached my office or my destination, out of the pollution of the roads and the city streets, I just dab a cotton wool dab and cleanse my face and hands. That immediately refreshes me, and gives my skin a golden glow. And also, there is just this faint exotic hint of marigolds as a fragrance and scent.

- I once made a paste of marigolds, and put them up on a cut. It was very soothing and healed it well. And then I used a paste of turmeric and Marigold to remove the scar. This ointment can easily be made at home by washing marigolds well and pounding them freshly with turmeric to make a paste. This can then be applied to the mild cuts and bruises and then bandaged up.

My grandmother used to use this paste upon her accident prone kids and grandkids, but nowadays ladies are so fidgety and careful about hygiene, that they would spend lots of money using chemical antiseptics, when natural cures are in their gardens and kitchens.

How to Make Marigold Skincare Cream

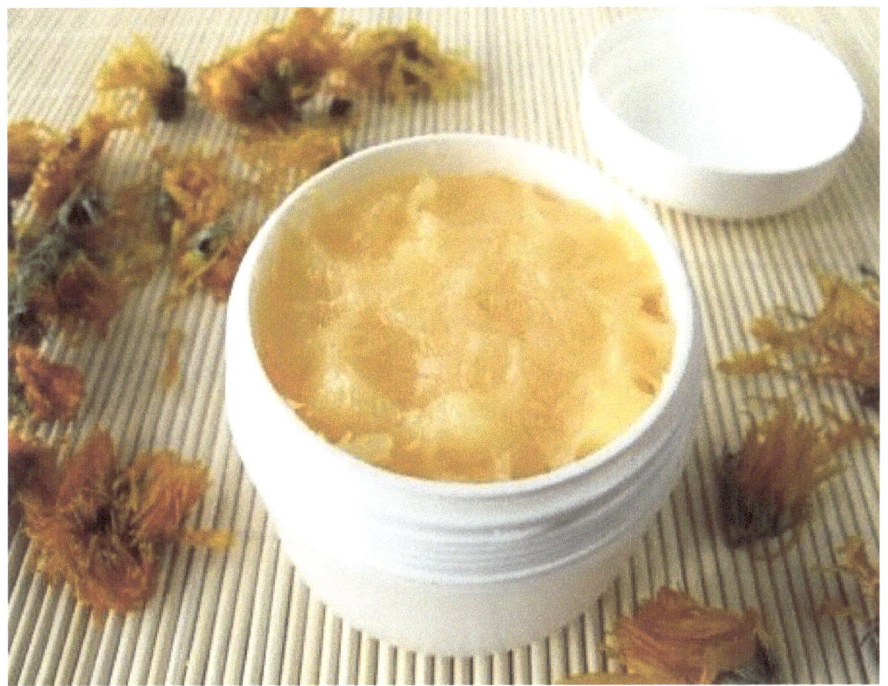

Marigold skin cream

You can either use Marigold   essential oils [read how to make essential oils in the appendix of this book] or you can use fresh Marigold   petals to make this exotic, natural skincare cream. Believe you me, this cream can keep you looking youthful, and because it has no chemical preservatives and it is completely natural, it is the much better to a much-hyped, very expensive and branded chemical beauty product out there with chemical-based products like parabens, Ubiquinone , Retinyl Palmitate, Cetearyl Olivate and Sorbitan Olivate in them.

Remember that the base for every good rejuvenating skin cream is almond oil and beeswax. Their proportions depend on how creamy or how thick you want the cream to be. Too much, Doyle will make your cream rather "watery "and too much beeswax will make it solid and chunky.

Melt the beeswax and the almond oil together in a pan placed in another pan with hot water. Once I could not find beeswax easily available in the market, so I used coconut oil, because after all, I was using this homemade cream on my own skin. Also, I placed this cream in the fridge so that I did not have to add a preservative, which you can do further on in the recipe.

Next step – boil the Marigold   petals in 1 cup of water. You may strain it. Now slowly and steadily add the boiled water – petal mixture to the beeswax and almond oil mixture while whisking it thoroughly. Let the emulsifying process takes place slowly. Just imagine that you are making mayonnaise, when the emulsifying oil is added, drop by drop to the eggs and mustard while whisking. The same process works here. When everything is of a required creamy consistency, you can add the preservatives. Well, I never do that, but you would want to.

Add the preserving chemicals – Sodium benzoate and lactic acid at a ratio of 20 mls lactic acid to 5g sodium benzoate (1/2 tsp). These are readily available at a chemists or a drugstore. Being in India, I added Rosewater to this mixture. You can either get this in the market or you can make your own Rosewater. [Recipe given in the appendix.]

I went a bit further, I chopped up fresh Marigold, rose and jasmine petals finely and added them to my calendula cream to give just that hint of exotic natural fragrance and daintiness. Do you know that this cream is wonderful for skincare as well as for cuts, stings and burns too?

I normally use Marigold   essential oil to prepare skincare creams and use the water for lotions.

Using Marigold And Hibiscus For Hair Care

Do you know that the gypsies in India use dried Marigold   and hibiscus petals in their natural egg and fuller salt shampoos to keep their hair lovely? They also add these petals to coconut oil and used it as a natural moisturizer.

Marigolds in Cooking

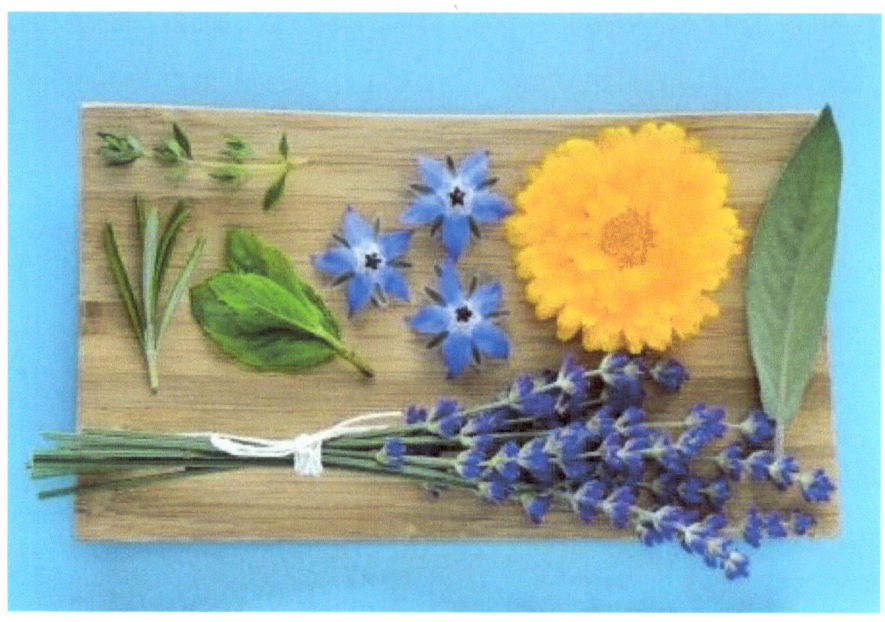

Summer herbs and edible flowers – herbs include Thyme, Rosemary, Mint, borage (borago) , Marigold   (Calendula officinalis), Salvia and Lavender (Lavandula)

One of my French gourmet chef friends said that she regularly used Marigold   petals and nasturtium leaves in her salads to add the last cachet of style and color to her dishes.

She is not the only one who knows that marigolds, nasturtiums, chive flowers and dandelions are really delicious. So even though Middle Eastern, Chinese, Asian, including Indian cuisine has been using flowers in cookery for millenniums, it is nice to see that the West is finally waking up to the fact, that many flowers are healthy, flowers are beautiful, and flowers are edible. But remember that not all flowers are edible. Also, any flowers which have been subjected to pesticides may harm you. Do not harvest any plants, which are growing by the roadside. Just imagine all the pollutants which have been incorporated in a plant, ever since it saw the light of day by the side of the Highway.

Also, another major rule-f lowers when edible should be used sparingly. You never know when somebody's delicate digestive system may say, hey, this dish was delicious and a sensory miracle, but it is playing havoc with my digestive system. If you have somebody in the family with this sort of system, do not experiment with marigolds or other flowers in cooking. However, if all of them have constitutions of ostriches and also enjoy innovative cooking, why not take a chance and garnish some of your dishes with nasturtium leaves and Marigold petals. Add some zing to soups, pasta or rice dishes, herb butters, and salads. These Petals can also add a yellow tint to soups, spreads, and scrambled eggs.

Wash the petals thoroughly and dry before you chop them up.

Here is one of my favorite recipes for making **Marigold butter along with herbs.**

For this, I go crazy. I pick up all my favorite herbs like Sage, parsley, thyme, marjoram, and even garlic, bishops, we weed, red chilies, rock salt, pepper, cumin seed, aniseed and anything else upon which I can lay my hands. Let me admit that I love butter! And herbal butter. That is better! You may also want to add chives and other herbs to this mixture, because after all, all of them are natural, all of them are delicious, and all of them are adding taste to butter.

1 pound sweet unsalted butter, at room temperature. Mix all the chopped herbs and well powdered spices well into this butter. Now add some finely

chopped Marigold   petals into this butter mixture. I normally place it in a cool place overnight so that all the goodness of the herbs and spices soak into the butter. Then I place the herbal butter in a glass bottle and refrigerate. Yummy. It lasted for six months and more with me, but a friend told me that her family finished it up in eight days, spreading this butter over every visible edible surface. Well, that is your prerogative!

Please remember that you are choosing the right Marigold to eat. This is what it is – Signet Marigold , also known as Tagetes tenuifolia (aka T. signata). So, you may ask a more experienced gardener about the Marigold   you want to sow in your garden, if you want to use it in cooking. But if you want to use Marigold   only for beauty preparations, all the different varieties are going to suit your purpose perfectly.

Rice is one of the most popular dishes in Asia, eaten extensively in India, China, Thailand, Malaysia, and so on. That is the reason why rice dishes are integral parts of oriental cuisine.

This recipe is for spiced liver with rice – with the Indian touch.

6 ounces long grain rice –basmati for choice.

4 onions peeled and chopped

1 tablespoon ginger garlic mixture – minced

2 tablespoons oil

2 tablespoons finely chopped Marigold petals and ¼ teaspoon turmeric.

Two level teaspoons – a mixture of spices like dried coriander, cloves and cardamom.

¾ Pint water.

15 to 20 raisins

Salt and Black Pepper

Spicy Liver –

500 g lamb liver.

1 teaspoon apple cider vinegar, and if you have Worcestershire sauce around, that is even better to give it the piquant flavor.

2 teaspoons flour

2 teaspoons ground coriander

1 teaspoon rocksalt.

2 tablespoons oil

Chop the liver into bite-size pieces and sprinkle with vinegar/sauce

Heat the oil in a saucepan. Add the onion and crushed garlic, fry gently till the onion is soft and brown.

Rinse the rice in a strainer under cold running water so that the extra starch is removed. Add the rice to the anion and garlic mixture, and then add all the other ingredients like petals, spices, turmeric, water, raisins and rock salt. You may also want to add some pepper if you want.

Bring to a boil and stir well.

Reduce the heat to a simmer. Cover the pan with a lid and allow the rice to be cooked for 12 to 15 minutes. This rice is going to be cooked well when all the water is absorbed.

Season the flour with coriander, pepper and half teaspoons salt and toss the liver in it to coat. Fry liver in all, gently over medium heat for 3 to 4 minutes until it is slightly crisped. Remember that frying over high heat, and for a longer period of time is going to make the liver leathery. Well cooked liver always looks brownish pink in the inside. Serve with spiced rice.

Did you know that apart from ancient cookery, medieval cookery also used Marigold extensively in making sweetmeats?

So if you want a unique **Apple Marigold tart**, here is the recipe.

10 ml petals from marigolds. – 3- 4 tablespoons minced Marigold petals at the most.

1 cooking apple, peeled and cored

200g ricotta cheese

6 egg yolks

2 tbsp butter

1/4 tsp ground mace, and other spices. The Elizabethans found it difficult to get spices, but their modern descendants can use cloves, cinnamon, cardamoms and other spices you have in your kitchen closet.

One pie crust – (see Appendix.)

Combine the peeled, chopped and diced – once I minced it – apple and 2 tbsp water in a small pan. Bring to a simmer and cook, uncovered, for about 20 minutes or until the apple has broken down. Add the flower petals to the apple along with the butter and spices. Now, puree it in a beater/mixer. Also, beat the cream cheese in a bowl until soft. Add the egg yolks to the cream cheese and beat until combined. Now work in the apple and Marigold   mix. This is our custard filling.

Turn this mixture into the blind-baked pastry shell then transfer to an oven pre-heated to 180 degrees C and bake for about 25 minutes, or until the pastry is golden and the custard filling has set. This can be served either hot or cold.

For all those people who are just going to say, hey DJ, just stop being such a tiresome know it all and what is blind baked? Well, blind baked is the term normally used by bakers who make pie crusts beforehand, and preserve them. And then when they need to make pies, all they do is take out a pie crust from the nearest refrigerator, fill with filling, bake and serve. I must admit that I very rarely make pie pastry when I can get it so easily from the friendly neighborhood baker!

Appendix

How to extract essential oils from fresh plucked Marigold petals

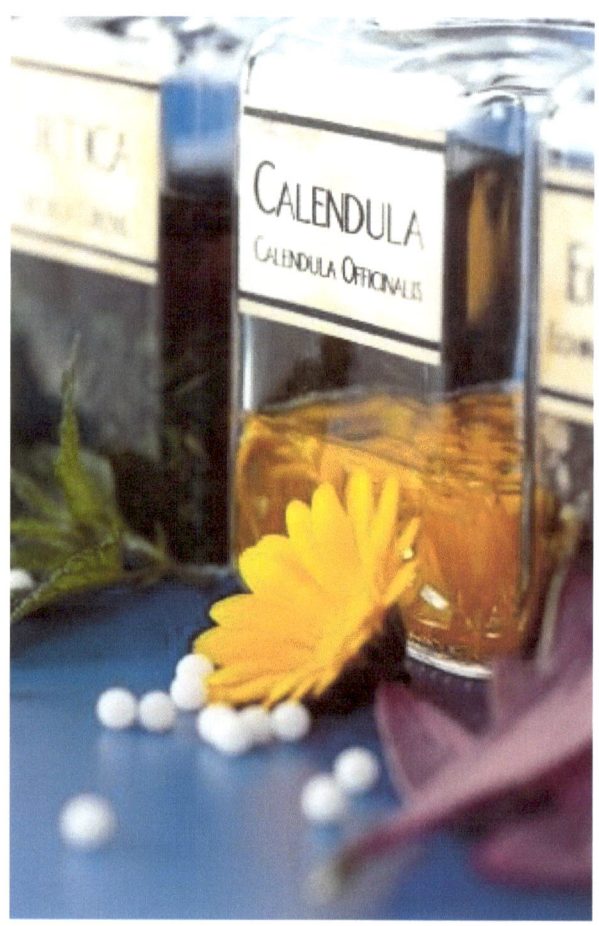

Calendula oil extract

For this method, you need to have a large supply of orange gold, and yellow Marigold petals, and lots of ice handy. Fresh Marigold flowers are best because dried Marigold flowers are good for seed, but I have not found them as powerful a source of essential oils as a fistful of fresh petals. Make sure that no calyx or green portion of the flower is mixed with the petals.

Take a large cooking pot, insert a clean brick or rock in its bottom, fill the pot with Marigold petals ,-the more the merrier, and red and orange flowers for choice. If you have picked them early in the morning that is really good, because that is the time when the aroma is strongest. No hybrids please.- around the brick. Cover with water and place a small glass dish on top of the brick.

Put a stainless steel bowl on top of the pot and fill with ice. Simmer about three hours depending how many petals you have, replacing the ice as needed. The bowl with the ice will condense the steam which will then drip down into the glass bowl. The water in the glass bowl is your Marigold water, which I normally use as a wonderful skin toner and cleanser and on top will be a pure layer of oil. This is the essential oil. You can separate these and use the water as a beauty product and the oil in all your beauty preparations.

Here is another quicker method for all those people who are strapped for time –

For this, you will have to have all the petals as well as a vegetable oil ready. 1 1/2 cups of vegetable oil and 250 grams of petals gave me 1 1/2 cups of infused oil.

• Place half of the Marigold petals and all the oil in a container with a tight lid.

- Put a container in a pan, fill the pan up with water to within 1 inch of the top of the container and simmer this slowly for 2 hours. This water bath makes sure that your precious oil is exposed to prolonged heating without spoiling the oil by burning or boiling. To save time and energy costs, I normally boil 2-3 airtight containers together.

- After two hours, allow the mixture to cool slightly and then strain it well. Now, we are just halfway through the process and the infusion has changed color. At this strength, this infusion is mild enough to use as baby oil or bath oil. Refill the canister with the remaining Marigold petals, cover with the strained oil and return to the water bath. Simmer gently for another two hours. Don't forget to replace the lid! Also make sure to check the water level to make sure that the water has not boiled away completely. Nobody has any use for burnt oil.

When the oil has cooked enough, pour it through a muslin cloth or very fine strainer. If you are using fresh petals, there might be some watery liquid at the bottom of the oil. Remember to separate out this liquid and throw it away, because it is quite certain to spoil the oil if it is left unattended.

Once the oil has been strained , gather all the petals in the cloth and wring them out to extract every drop of oil . This oil will keep fresh for a year but it will eventually become rancid. Many cosmetologists thus add some wheat germ oil to delay the spoiling process -- (about 25 g.)

As for the spent petals, I do not throw them away, but I put them into my bathwater so as not to waste them! These oils have to be poured into clean bottles. Remember to store them away in dark and not transparent bottles in a cool and dark place away from the sunlight.

I also found this oil getting rancid if I did not shake it often, and straining it, if there was any sort of brownish deposit at the bottom of the bottle and also if it was kept in the sun. So remember that wheat germ oil, as well as the cool dark place for storage is a good idea.

How to make Rose water

Rosewater is normally available in European and American markets at exorbitant prices,- but in India , in other parts of Asia and the Middle East too-, anybody with access to the red rose – Rosa Damascena and a little bit of free time , can enjoy making Rosewater at home. This Rosewater is used in cosmetics, as well as in cookery to impart the flavor of the Rose to your meal or to your skin.

Ingredients needed-

1 Cup Rose petals – 12 to 14 flowers.

2 cups water

Lots of ice.

A huge cooking pan – pan number one – with lid in which another pan – pan number two – can be placed comfortably.

Rosewater is just a matter of distillation. Put a wire stand in pan number one, on which you are going to stand the other pan number two. The condensed Rosewater is going to fall into pan number two.

Place the petals at the bottom of the pan number one. Now, cover the petals with water. Place pan number two on the wire stand. Now take the lid and place it upside down on pan number one, thus effectively covering the Rose petals, pan number two and the water. The Rose water is going to condense when you place the blocks and chunks of ice on the inverted lid.

You are going to have a cupful of precious distilled Rosewater, after 25 minutes of slow steaming of the Rose petals.

Precautions – remember to have enough of water to cover the Rose petals. Also, it should not be of such a large quantity, that it displaces the wire stand.

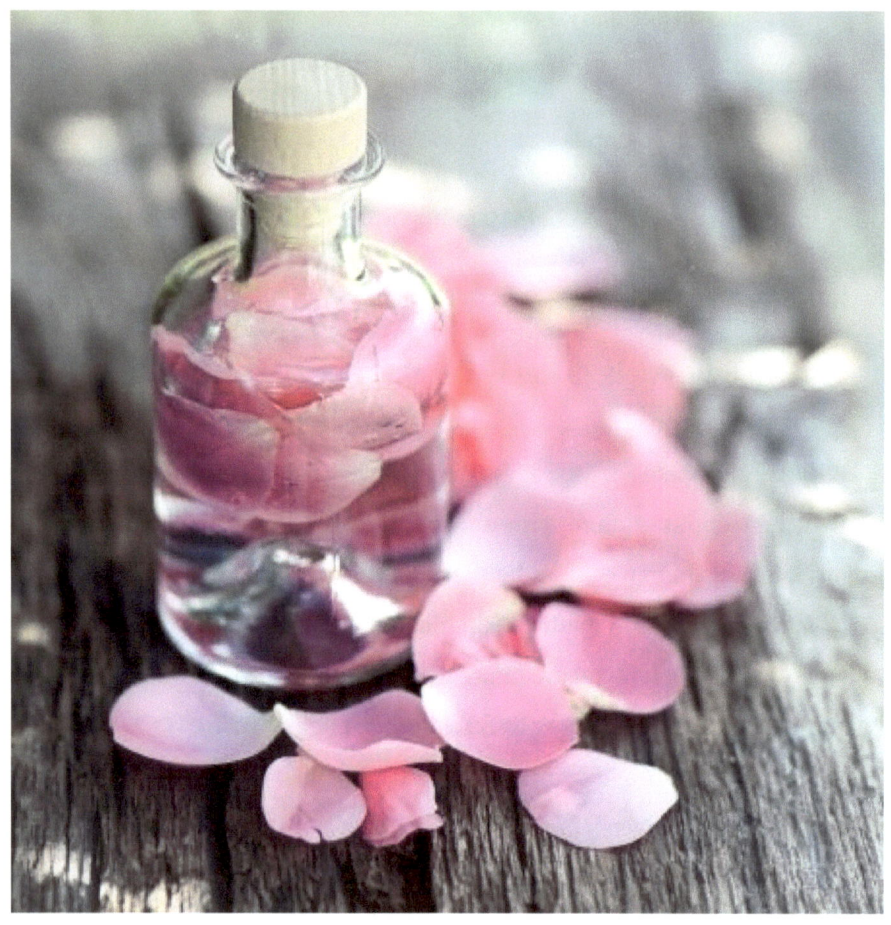

Rose water

This cooled water is now pure Rosewater. Placed it in a sterilized glass bottle. Use it to your hearts content. You may see a little bit of oil swimming over the surface of the water. This is Rose oil, and is even more precious. So if you used lots of petals in a larger pan, you may find even more Rose oil.

This method is for all those people who use a pressure cooker while cooking food. In fact, it is a common way to cook food in Indian kitchens, though I was surprised to see that many of my Australian friends were surprised on being confronted with a pressure cooker for the first time. Anyway, I digress.

You would need water, petals, a pressure cooker and a long thin pipe which it does not melt, when subjected to heat.

Put the water and the petals in the pressure cooker and cover it. Now cover the thin pipe with wet cloth in order to keep it cool. Attach this pipe on the lid of the pressure cooker where you normally attach the weight. Allow the petals to cook slowly, they seem to build up, go through the cooled pipe and collect in a utensil. I tried this way too, but I find the ice on the lid one easier!

How to make pie crust

175g plain flour

1 egg yolk

3 tbsp (about) cold water

Dice the butter, add to the flour hen rub in with your fingertips until the mixture comes together and resembles fine breadcrumbs. Add the egg yolk and work into the flour and butter mix. Now add the remaining cold water, a little at a time, and work together until the mixture comes together as a dough. Cover this with clingfilm and chill in the refrigerator for 20 minutes before rolling and using.

Roll out the pastry and use to line a 22cm diameter deep pie dish. Line with greaseproof (waxed) paper ,fill with baking beans then transfer to an oven pre-heated to 180°C and blind bake for about 15 minutes, or until the pastry is just dry to the touch.

Remove from the oven, take out the paper and baking beans and set aside until ready for baking.

Conclusion

So now that you know all about the magic of marigolds, and how it can be used in beauty products and in cooking, have fun experimenting with this tenacious and beautiful flower. Chinese and Indian naturalists and herbalists have been stirring Marigold as a blood purifier for millenniums, even though Western scientists are still looking into this plant as a source of medicine. I am not giving you any blood purifying recipes using Marigold , because I am not a doctor. On the other hand, all the beauty preparations using Marigold have been made by me and I have been using them for decades. These are tried and tested. Also the Marigold dish recipes have been tried out by me. Yes, they are tasty. But remember, Do Not put handfuls of Marigold petals in your dishes, when cooking. But Do put handfuls of these petals in oils if you are making infusions.

Have fun with Marigolds.

Look out for more of our herbs and flowers books, giving you more information and knowledge about flowers, spices and other plants and all their natural health giving and beauty enhancing benefits.

Author Bio

Dueep Jyot Singh is a Management and IT Professional who managed to gather Postgraduate qualifications in Management and English and Degrees in Science, French and Education while pursuing different enjoyable career options like being an hospital administrator, IT,SEO and HRD Database Manager/ trainer, movie scriptwriter, theatre artiste and public speaker, lecturer in French, Marketing and Advertising, ex-Editor of Hearts On Fire (now known as Solctice) Books Missouri USA, advice columnist and cartoonist, publisher and Aviation School trainer, ex- moderator on Medico.in, banker, student councilor ,travelogue writer … among other things! One fine morning, she decided that she had enough of killing herself by Degrees and went back to her first love -- writing. It's more enjoyable! She already has 38 published academic and 14 fiction- in- different- genre books under her belt.

When she is not designing websites or making Graphic design illustrations for clients who want Walt Disney, Norman Rockwell , JJ Grandville or Hed Kandy type illustrations, she is busy browsing in old bookshops for antique books,-she has a mouthwatering collection of priceless First editions and rare books…including R.L. Stevenson, O.Henry, Dornford Yates, Maurice Walsh, C.N.Williamson, and the crown of her collection- Dickens "The Old Curiosity Shop," and so on… Just call her "Renaissance Woman" - collecting herbal remedies, making one of a kind creations in Irish Crochet and Aran knitting, acting like Universal Helping Hand/Agony Aunt, or escaping to her dear mountains for a bit of exploring, collecting herbs and plants , trekking, and rappelling.

Check out some of the other JD-Biz Publishing books

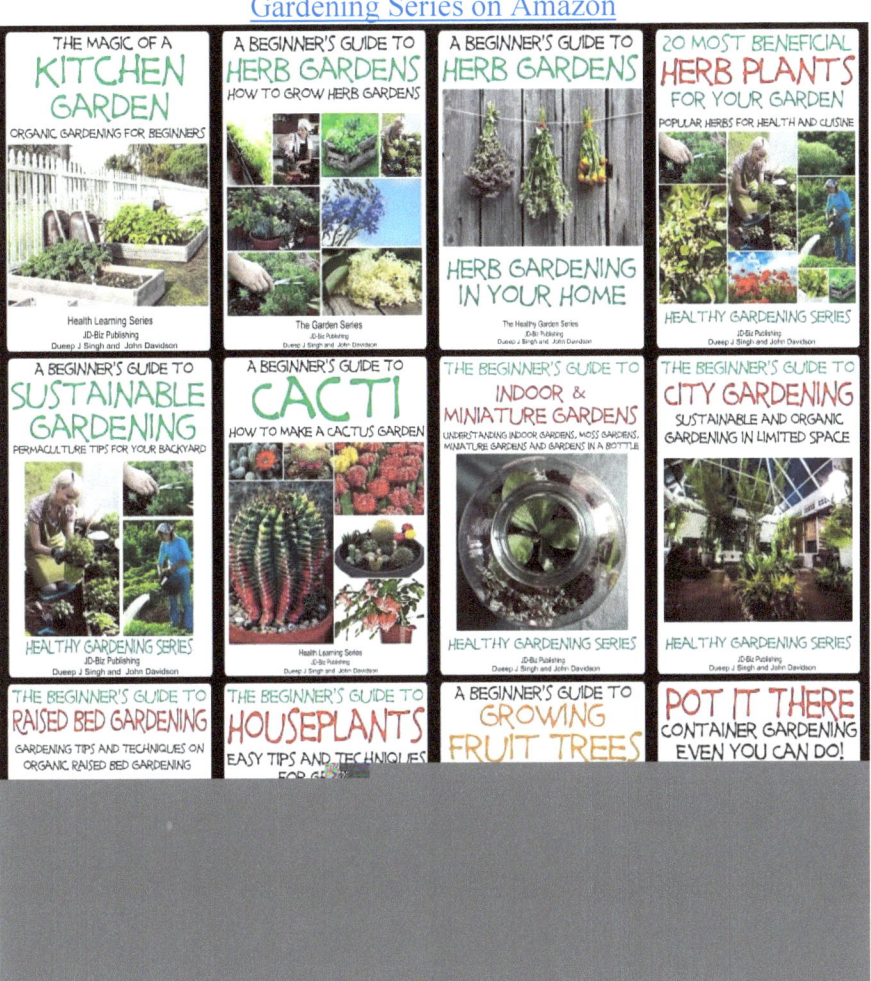

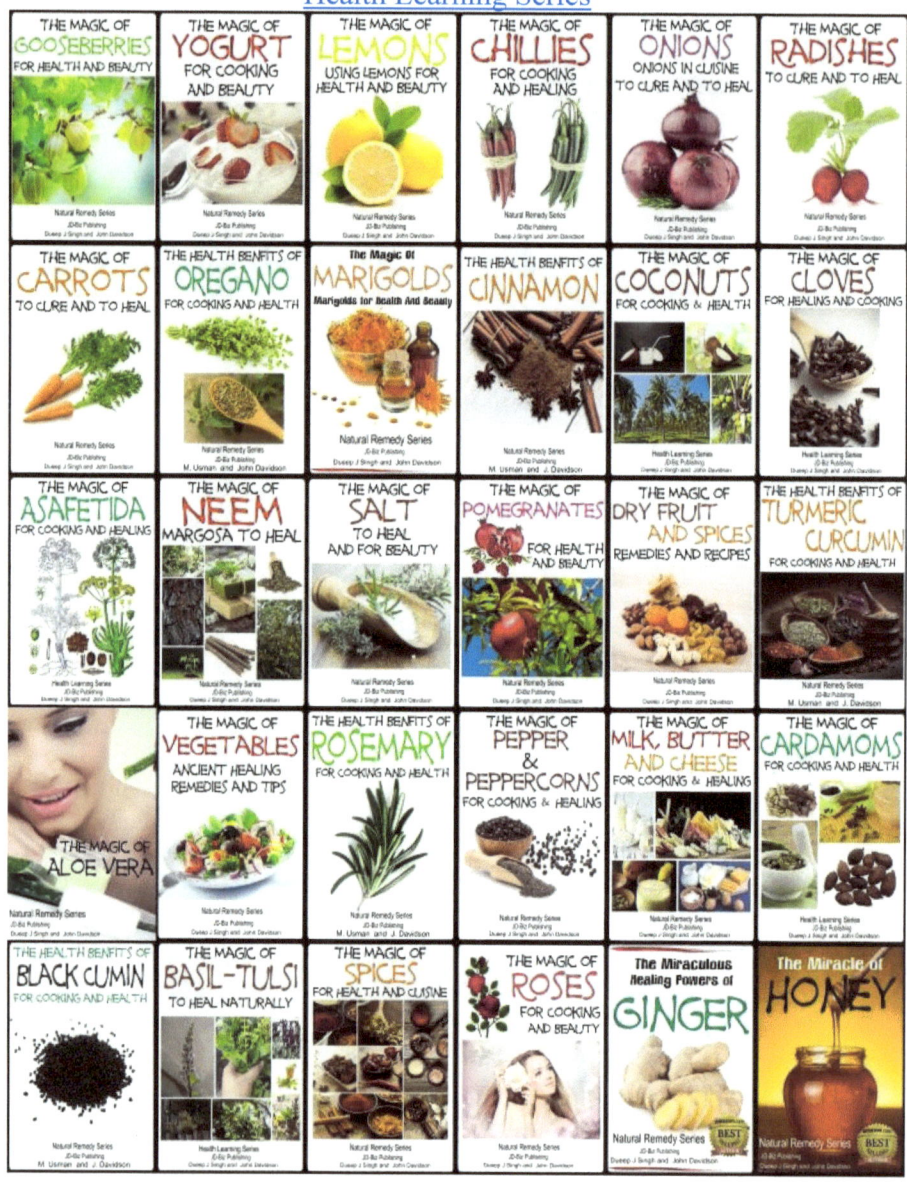

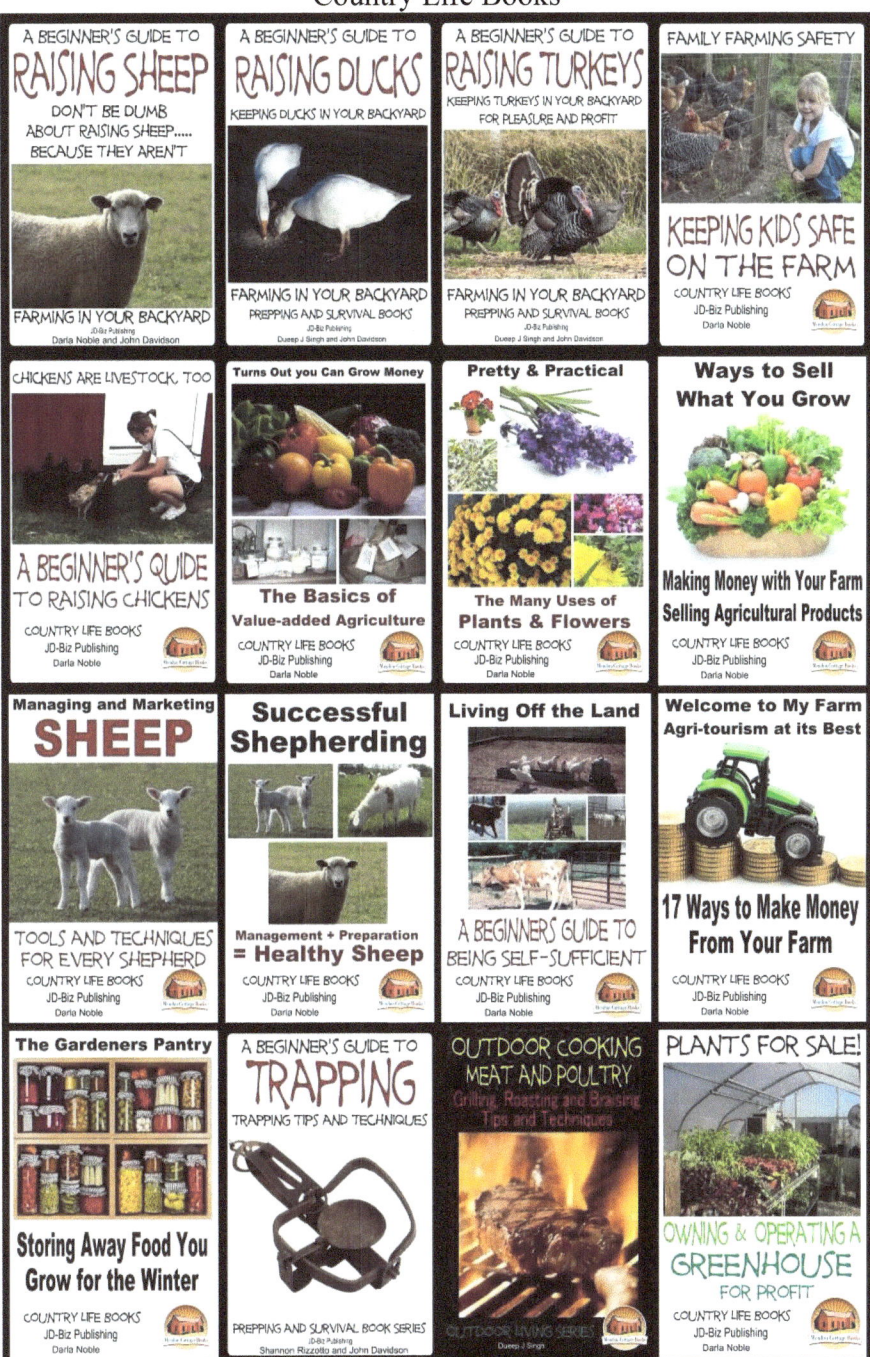

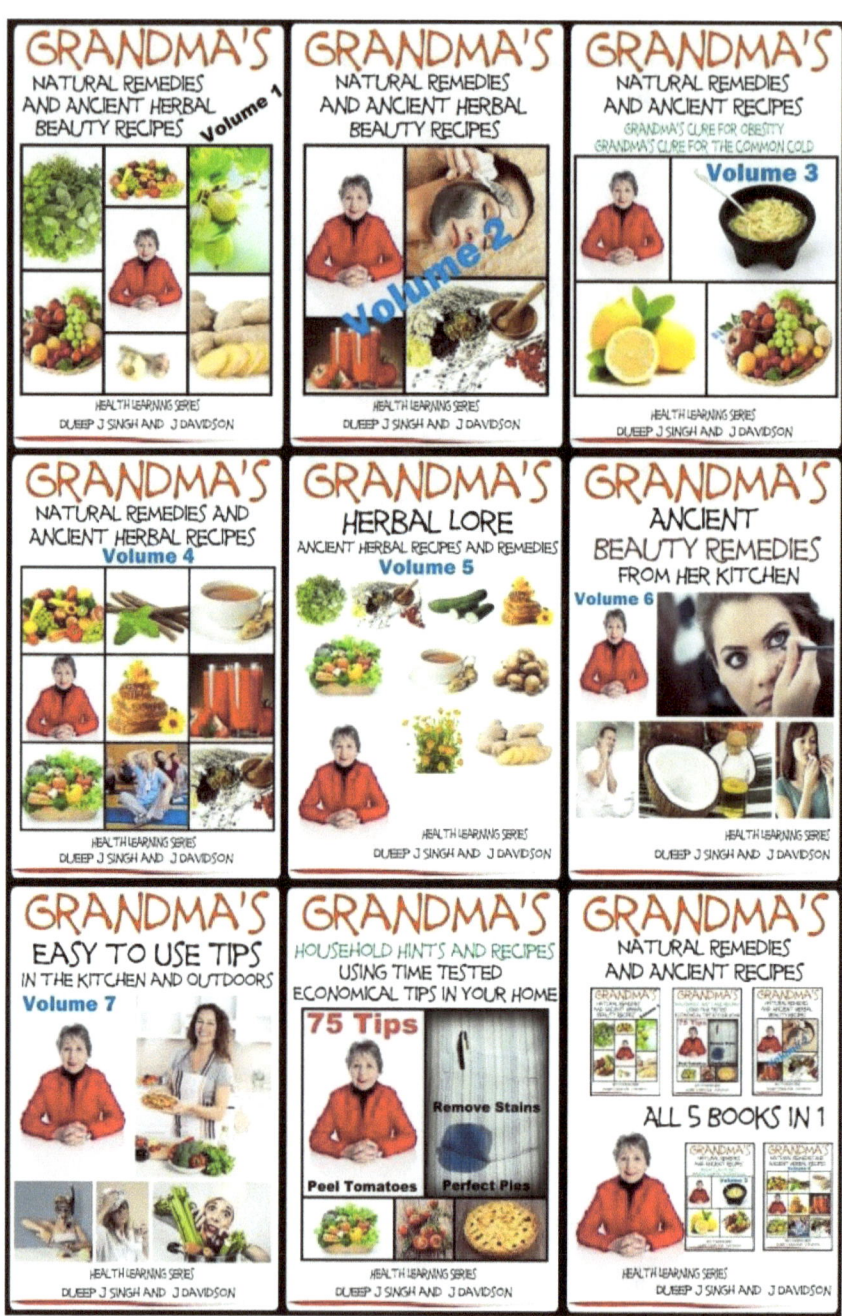

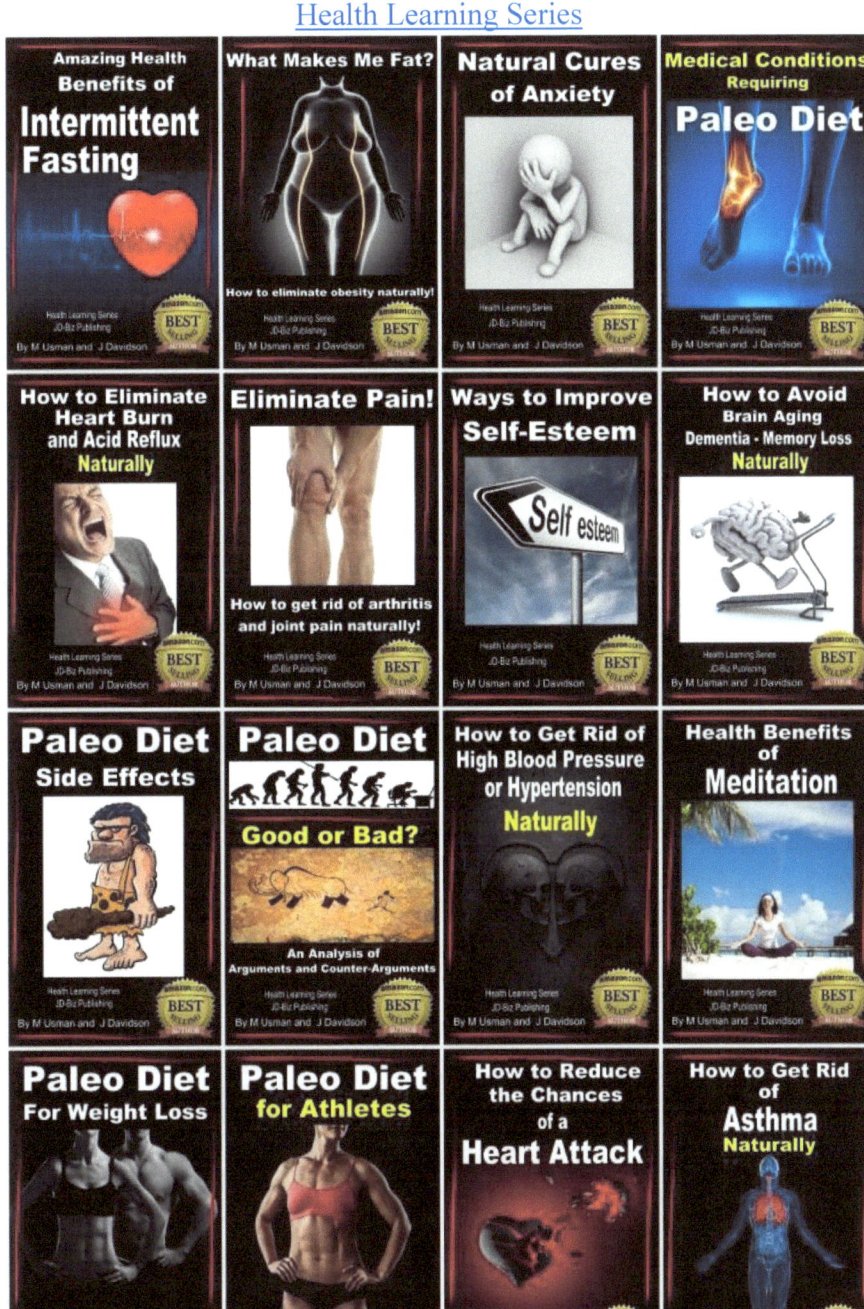

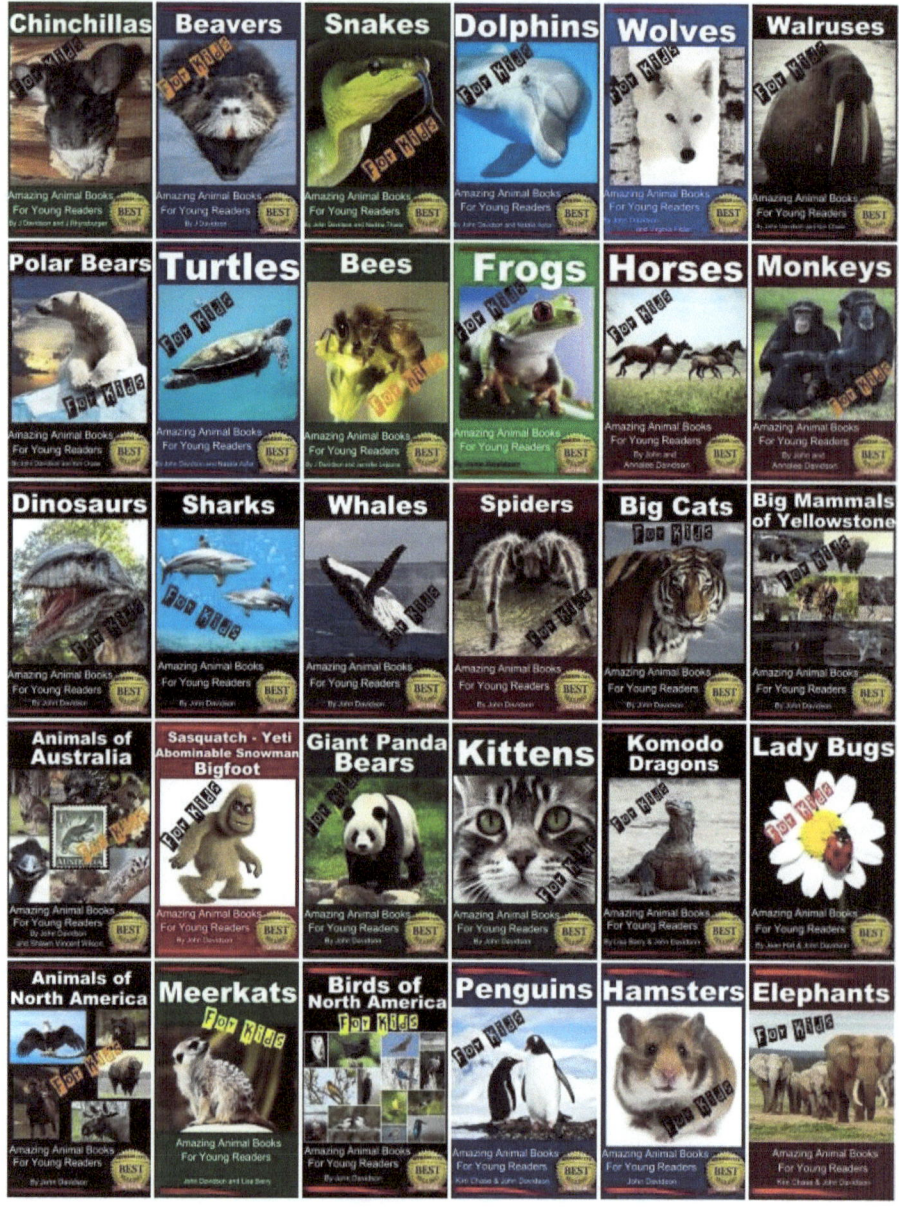

Learn To Draw Series

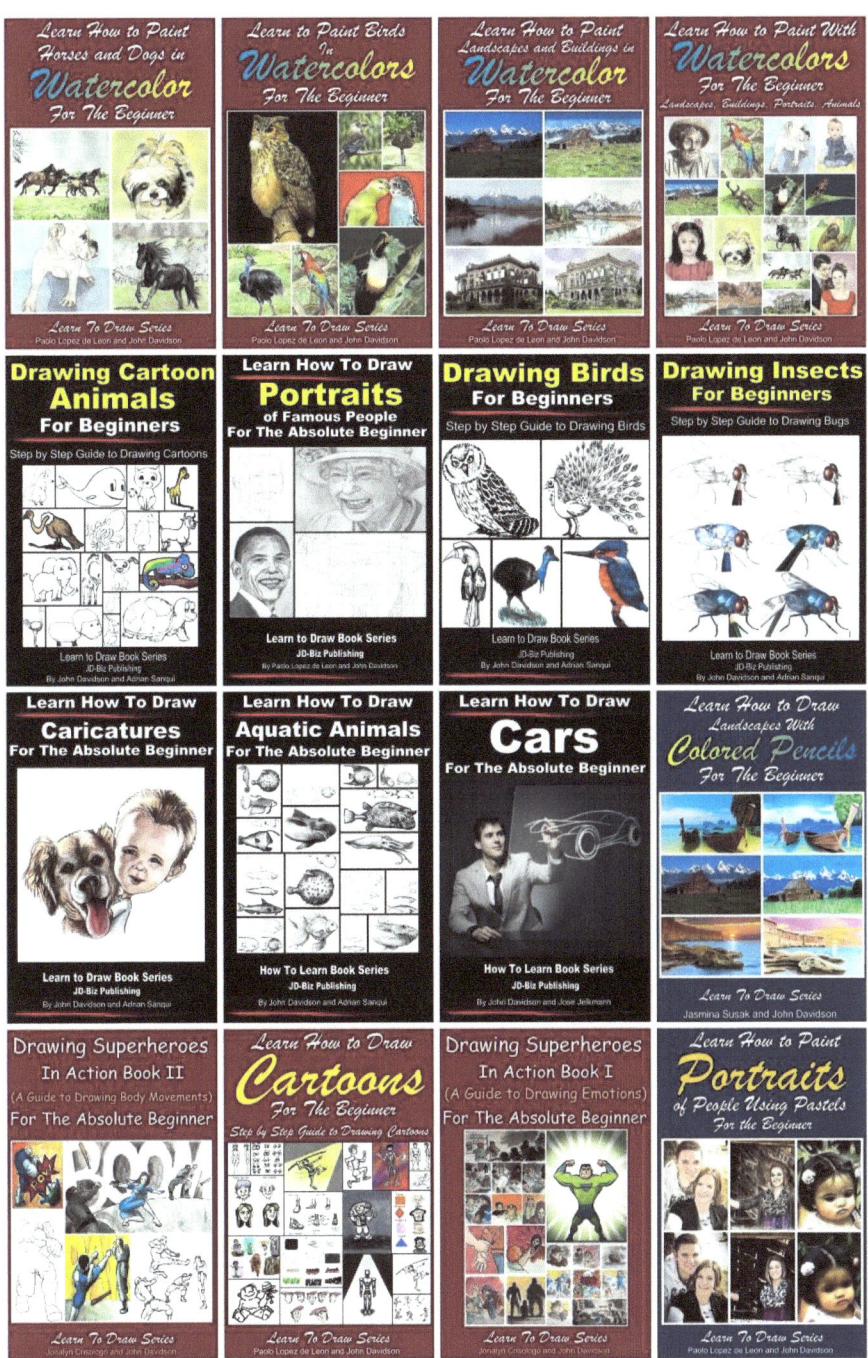

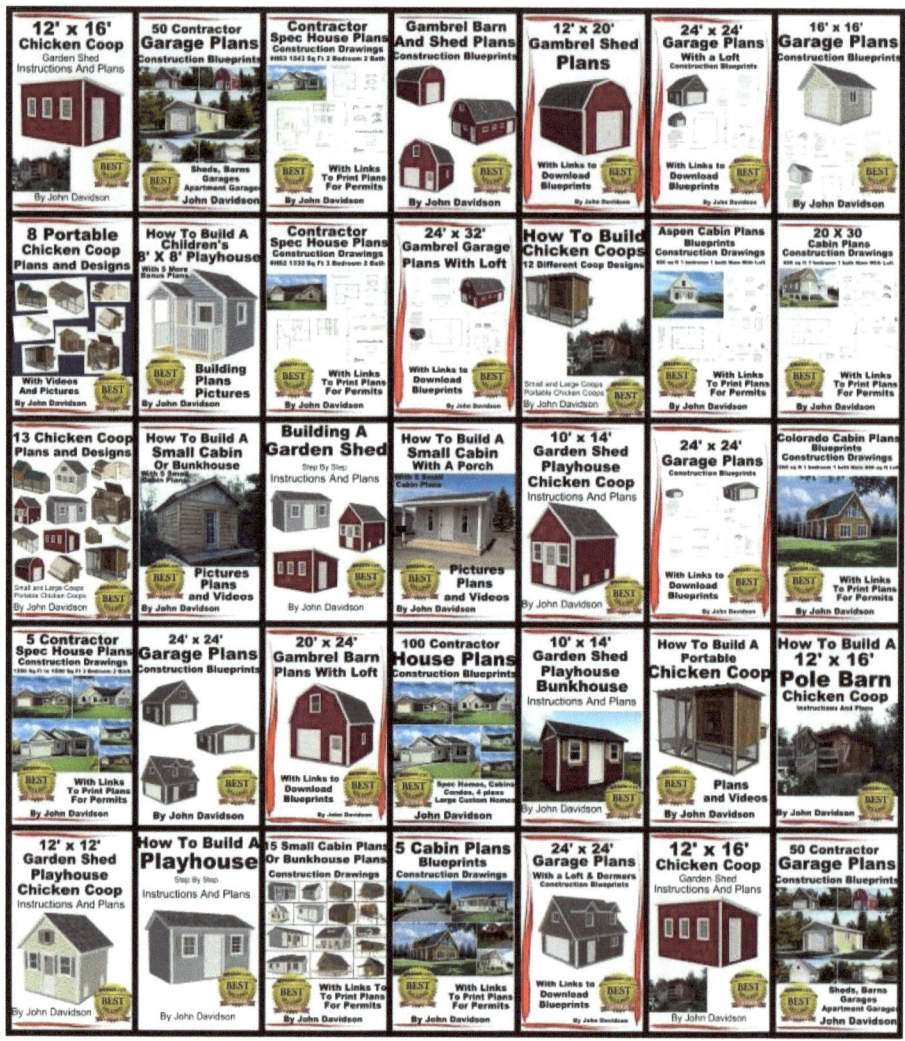

Entrepreneur Book Series

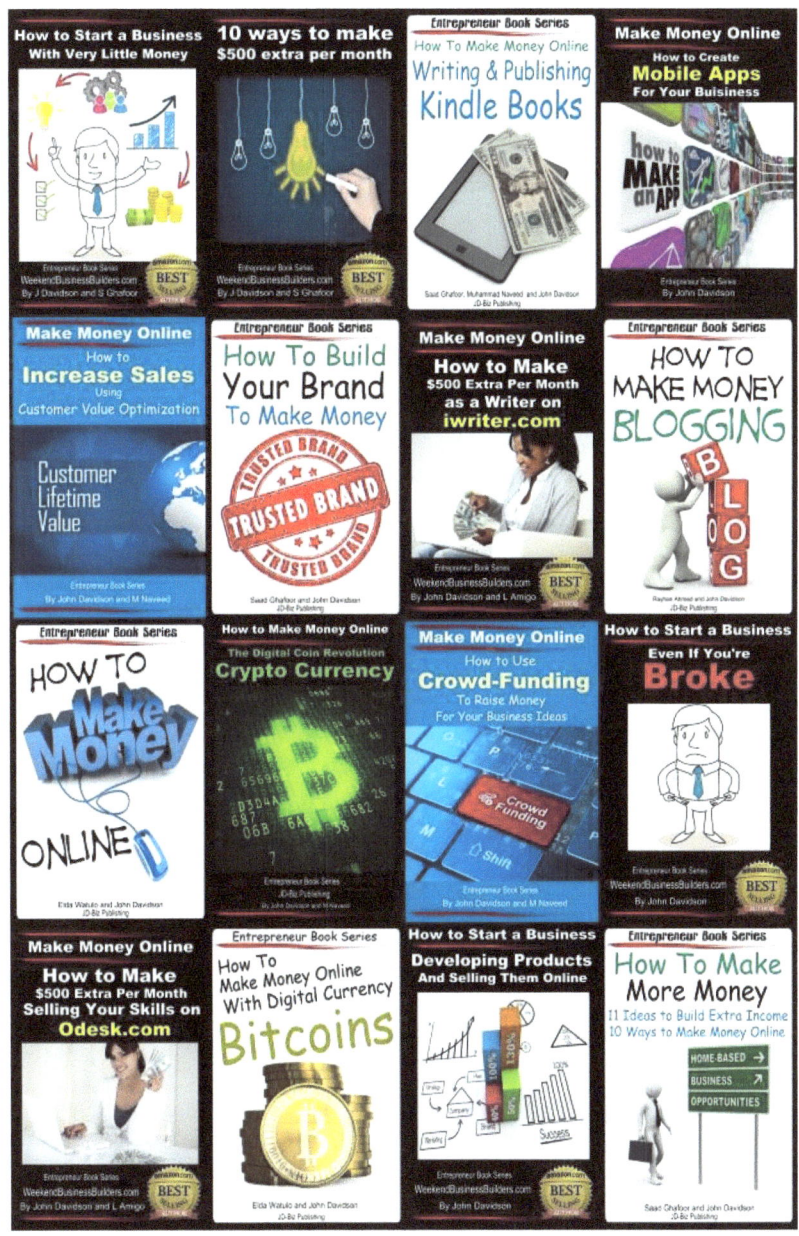

Our books are available at

1. Amazon.com
2. Barnes and Noble
3. Itunes
4. Kobo
5. Smashwords
6. Google Play Books

Download Free Books!

http://MendonCottageBooks.com

Publisher

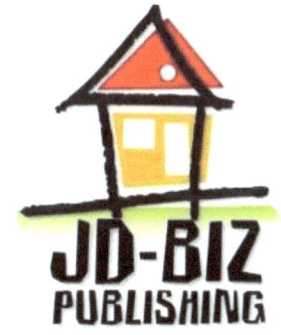

JD-Biz Corp

P O Box 374

Mendon, Utah 84325

http://www.jd-biz.com/

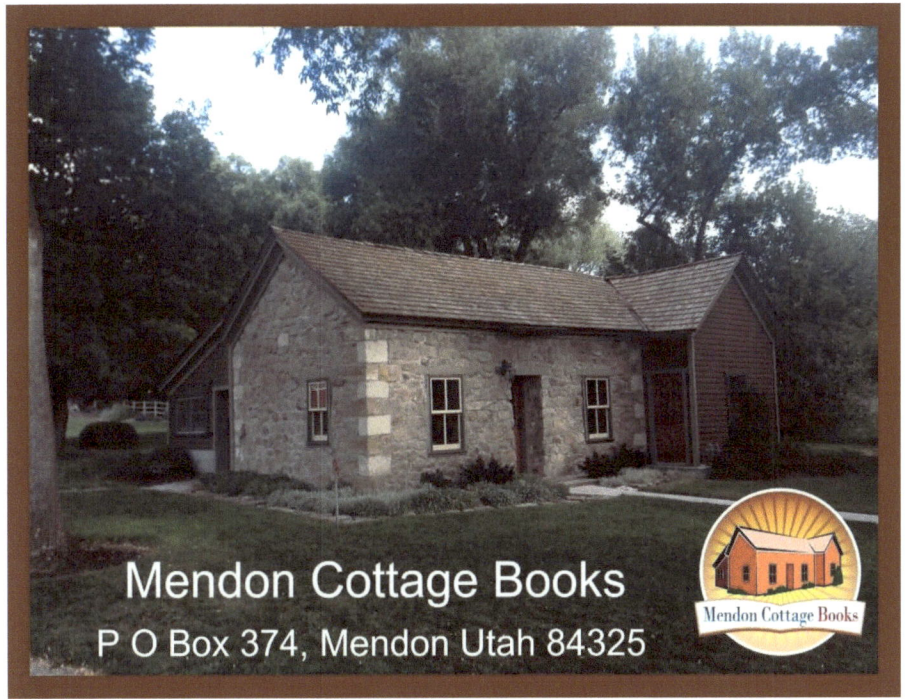